M000013249

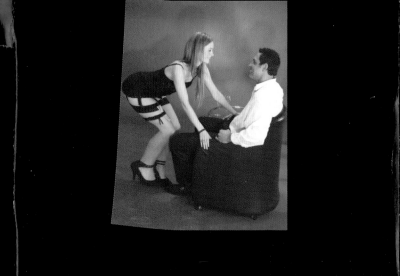

the little bit naughty book of
LAP DANCING
for your lover

the little *bit naughty* book of
LAP DANCING
for your lover

rebecca drury

Amorata Press

Text copyright © Rebecca Drury 2006
Photographs copyright © Alistair Hughes 2006
This edition copyright © Eddison Sadd Editions 2006

Rebecca Drury has asserted her right to be identified as the author
of this work under the Copyright, Designs and Patents Act 1988.

All rights reserved. No part of this publication may be reproduced, stored in a retrieval
system or transmitted in any form or by any means electronic, mechanical, photocopying
or otherwise without the prior written permission of the copyright owners.

Published in the U.S. by
Amorata Press,
an imprint of Ulysses Press
P.O. Box 3440
Berkeley, CA 94703
www.amoratapress.com

1 3 5 7 9 10 8 6 4 2

First published in the U.K. in 2006 as *Lap Dancing: The Naughty Girl's Guide*
by Connections Book Publishing Limited

Library of Congress Control Number 2006926000
ISBN-10: 1-56975-558-2
ISBN-13: 978-1-56975-558-7

AN EDDISON • SADD EDITION
Edited, designed, and produced by
Eddison Sadd Editions Limited
St Chad's House, 148 King's Cross Road
London WC1X 9DH
www.eddisonsadd.com

Phototypeset in Myriad using QuarkXPress on Apple Macintosh
Printed in Singapore

Distributed by Publishers Group West

Please note: The author, publisher and packager cannot accept any responsibility for
injury resulting from the practice of any of the dance moves set out in this book. Please
consult a professional if you are in doubt about any aspect of your health.

contents

introduction

I have danced all over the world, for thousands of people. I loved my job, but it wasn't until I fell in love and used my skills to entertain my partner that I truly realized the potency and joy of the experience. Since then, I've been on a mission to write this book.

I've now danced for my lover many times, and I would like to share with you the knowledge I've gained so that you may enjoy the same fantastic experience with your man.

You are about to discover a dance style that's influenced by many different forms of erotic dance. It's crucial that you have a strong sense of self-belief, so I've also drawn on aspects of the theatre and magic, to give you a highly charged confidence boost. I want you to dazzle your lover!

The first part of this book, Preparation, will provide all kinds of ideas to help you plan your big night. If you take the time to fully prepare yourself, your space and your partner, you should find that everything runs smoothly, and you'll be able to relax and enjoy yourself just as much as him!

There is so much more to erotic dancing than moving around sexually. In the next section, Style Matters,

you'll gain an insight into the psychology and performance of the dance. You'll realize the importance of eye contact and how to use your face and body to direct your lover' focus to exactly where you want it at any given moment. Now, *that's* power!

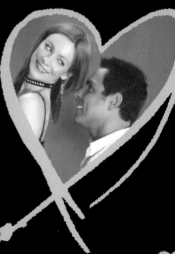

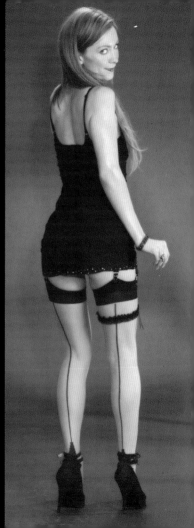

Once you've mastered the style, you'll be ready for Dance Moves, where you'll learn some of the classic erotic movements that you would see in any lap dancing club. Get these right and you'll have your lover transfixed from the moment you enter the room to the second you wave goodbye!

Of course, you'll want to put these moves together. The next section, The Unveiling, contains a dance routine demonstrating how to use the moves. It also shows you how to undress erotically as you dance. However, don't just follow my ideas. I'm here to guide you, but try to create some sensual dance moves of your own, too. Dancing in front of a mirror is a great way to see what looks good and, the more you do this, the more confident you'll become.

The final part of the book, The Fantasy, suggests ways to add even more fun to your show. Fantasy plays an important role, and many dancers take on a new persona when they perform. Find out how to create your own fantasy character and meet Phoenix, who's been with me in many a dance!

Erotic dance is self-expression, sometimes storytelling in movement, and always provocative.

With this book you can create a fabulous way to dance elegantly and erotically for your man. There is a spirit, a state of mind, that you must try to embrace before you embark on your first show. To understand and achieve this, I recommend that you read the whole book first.

Finally, never forget the most important principle behind this exotic dance style – enjoy yourself. Remember that it's your special night in as well as your lover's. Try to relax, and have a fabulous time.

preparation

Please believe me when I say that preparation and style are more important than being a brilliant dancer. Your lover will appreciate your dancing whatever you do, within reason, as long as he feels confident that you really want to perform for him.

The way to make him believe this is to put a little thought into creating the right atmosphere. Show him that it means a lot to you that you both enjoy the night. This section will give you all the information you need about planning a time and a place, and transforming yourself into a goddess …

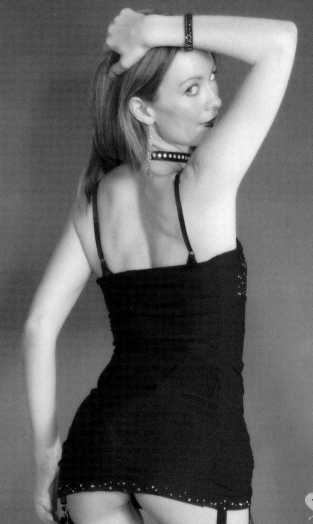

Making a date with your lover for the occasion is vital. If you surprise him when he's tired or not in the mood, it could ruin everything. Besides, he will want to relish the experience fully.

Set the date for a time when you'll both be feeling energetic and relaxed. By giving him a little advance warning, you'll be whetting his appetite with suspense and intrigue – the anticipation of meeting this new woman in his life will be worth every second of the wait!

Let your lover help you prepare for the show. Maybe he could compile a CD of some of your favourite music, or help you choose special lighting. The more you create the scene in his mind's eye, the more seriously he will take the evening.

Don't tell him what you're going to wear, though!

12

Dancing for a lover is a bonding ritual; a display of female sexuality that's enticing and flirtatious, not pornographic or promiscuous. It's a deeply profound act of spirituality and love.

All rituals are carried out in a sacred space. Before you dance, prepare the room, or the area, that you'll use. You could ask your partner to participate in this, as well. Make sure the space is clean and tidy. Surround yourselves with all your favourite things – fresh fruit to sweeten your palates, chocolate, champagne on ice.

Flowers with strong sexual characteristics, such as lilies or orchids, are subliminal aphrodisiacs, and will create a wonderful atmosphere. And rose petals sprinkled on the floor look and smell lovely. But the two of you must choose whatever will make this a great erotic night in for you – every couple is different. Let your imagination fly. Build a Bedouin tent, a den of iniquity, a fairy-tale castle, the Garden of Eden …

I always make sure there's a glass of water ready to drink if I get thirsty during the dance. There are also a few other things you can do with water, which I'll explain later!

Seating

Allocate a particular seating area for your lover. Make sure he knows that that's where he must be sitting while you perform. Put the music you'll be dancing to where he can find it easily, and make sure the lighting in the room is just right, so that when you return to perform, you'll be comfortable and at ease.

Lighting

It's best not to dance in a bright white atmosphere. If possible, invest in some red or pink lights and maybe even some flashing ones. Candles and dimmed lights also work well. Bear in mind that some effects can have unwanted consequences: for example, ultraviolet light can make capped teeth look luminous, although it's useful for making the skin look smoother!

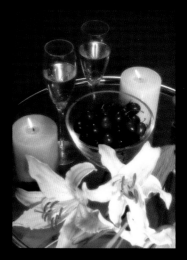

Blessings from Aphrodite

While you prepare the space, burn some incense and candles and say, or think, a small invocation to Aphrodite, goddess of love, beauty, passion and ecstasy. Focus on her and what she represents. Invite her to allow love, sex and romance into your life. Ask her to bless you with inner beauty and grace and to help you to inspire your lover with your dance.

Think of her just before your show begins, as well, and she will come to give you her support. Don't forget to thank her some time afterwards, too.

Final touches

Leave incense and candles burning throughout your performance if you can, to create a heady atmosphere and to help transport you both to other realms of consciousness.

Oh, and don't forget to unplug the telephone and put a 'Do Not Disturb' sign on the door!

On the evening of your date, ask your lover to entertain himself for a while so you can get ready. Make him wait just a little longer.

Your metamorphosis

Never let your man see you making the transformation from girl-next-door to goddess. Treat this as another ritual; one that's devoted to adornment and feeling like a movie star. Cover your body with beautiful oils and a little perfume. Gently massage yourself as you rub in the creams and lotions. This will help you to relax and focus.

Make sure you shave, leaving nothing to spill out of that G-string, especially at the back, girls! If you're feeling pale, think about getting a fake tan. You could try rougeing your nipples with a smudge of lipstick to emphasize them. Make your lover drool at the thought of them in his mouth.

As you turn yourself into this beautiful creature, you are creating a cloak of confidence. Use body glitter and lots of exotic make-up. Paint your nails and style your hair differently – wear it curled, straightened or crimped,

16

perhaps, and let it flow freely. Be glamorous, be gorgeous, be a star!

Take off your watch and anything else you usually wear, such as a wedding or engagement ring. Cut out any labels in your outfit to take your partner away from reality. Any labels or familiar jewellery will lessen the impact of all your efforts.

First-night jitters

If you suffer from nerves before you perform, try this calming exercise: breathe in through your nose as slowly and as deeply as you can, hold your breath for ten seconds, then slowly breathe out through your mouth. Do this three times, then breathe normally again. Repeat if necessary.

The alcohol rules

Don't drink too much before or during your dance, as you'll risk looking ridiculous. It's also dangerous to dance in high heels when drunk – and high heels are a must! You can always have a glass or two of something after your show, when I'm sure your man will be pouring you anything you desire! Be intoxicating – not intoxicated!

Dressing up is a return to innocence. It reminds me of wonderful lost hours spent dressing up dolls when I was a child. Except this time it's you that you're dressing up. Let your imagination run away with you. Look for unusual costumes, sparkly outfits, naughty uniforms; you might customize some charity shop clothes with sequins and beads. The internet is a fabulous place to find great costumes.

Keep it simple

This is a flowing, slow and sensuous dance style that should look as effortless as possible. Your aim should be to transport your lover and yourself into a carefree hypnotic trance and to make your man believe that you're dancing on a cloud, in a mist of sensuality. So make sure your costume is easy to take off. If you do have difficulty removing something, don't drop out of character. Slowly sway, turning your back to him, then give your full attention to the problem. Don't giggle or panic.

Don't wear anything that will restrict your movements – no zips at the back or hooks

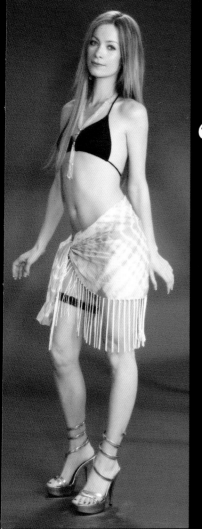

If you dance in stockings and suspenders, I strongly recommend that you leave them on throughout your dance; they'll look amazing. Wear your G-string over the top so you can take that off easily, if you wish!

(except in a bra), and only wear a corset if you intend to keep it on. Whatever you wear should be a breeze for you to remove. You shouldn't have to look down in order to undo something. Always practise getting out of your outfit beforehand.

For your first few dances, try wearing a short Lycra dress with beautiful underwear underneath, or a gorgeous bikini with a sarong. G-strings are the most flattering style of knickers, but they're not essential. If you wish to go nude, wear knickers that tie at the sides. It takes a great deal of skill and experience to remove the other kind!

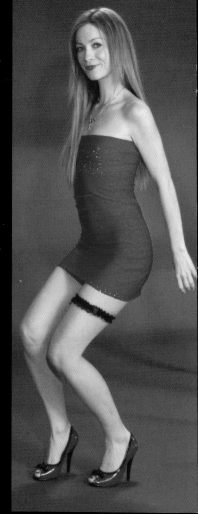

Attention to detail

Accessorize your outfit with lots of sparkly jewellery. There's nothing quite like seeing a lady topless or naked apart from some beautiful jewellery resting against her skin.

Take requests

Another must-have is high heels. Ask your partner beforehand whether he prefers shoes or boots. He may also have strong views about the colour and texture of your costume. Asking your lover for his opinion on these matters will help to build the sense of anticipation in his mind. However, you don't have to be guided by his views every time. Give him some surprises!

Be different

Dress any way you choose, as long as it's in a costume you would never normally wear. Be a nurse or a temple dancer, a goddess or a secretary; anything, but don't be yourself. When you change your clothes or your hair, you'll become a different woman in your man's eyes. Eventually you could build up a whole wardrobe of fantasy costumes!

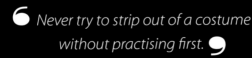

Never try to strip out of a costume without practising first.

21

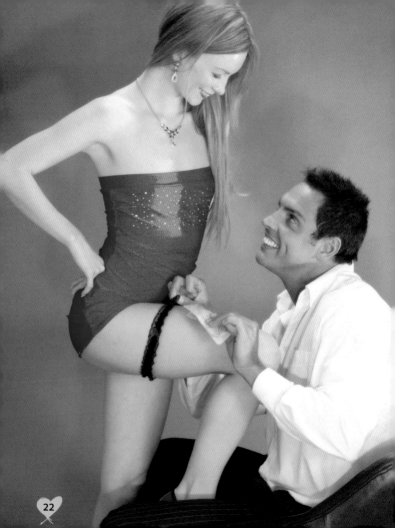

the garter

In my classes, I insist that all my students wear some money folded around a garter on their thigh. Why? Because it's a potent message that says you are worth paying for. It transforms you into a luxury item. The girls in the clubs with the most money in their garters get the most dances because it suggests they're good at what they do.

The garter is also a classic symbol of eroticism. It will help you to get into your new role. Who knows – if you're lucky, he may even take the hint and give you more money for a second show! If so, carry on the masquerade: tell him what you charge to go topless, fully nude and for hostessing – hostesses charge just to talk! Try to strike a deal with him.

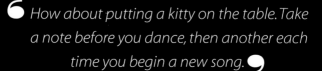

How about putting a kitty on the table. Take a note before you dance, then another each time you begin a new song.

making an entrance

You are now nearly ready to make your entrance. Use a phone to call your lover from outside the room. Using a gentle voice, ask him to put on your music. It should be loud enough to cover any creaking floorboards (or hip joints). If you're unable to use a phone, peep round the door to let him know you're ready. Talk to him, but don't let him see your costume.

Become someone new

Create the image of a fantasy character in your mind's eye. Imagining yourself bathed in the light and benevolence of Aphrodite, breathe deeply and try to invoke the magic of love, sex, inner beauty and grace. (For more about creating a fantasy character, see pages 88–9.)

If you have followed my instructions carefully, your man is going to be amazed.

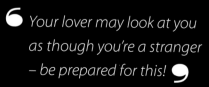

Your lover may look at you as though you're a stranger – be prepared for this!

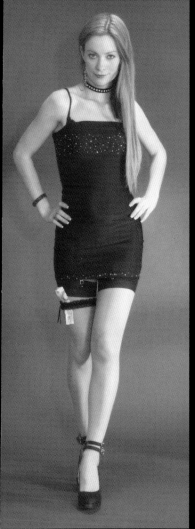

Be prepared for his jaw to drop and for him to look at you as though he doesn't know you. You will be a stranger to him – don't let this unsettle you. Brace yourself for his reaction, whatever it may be! It's up to you to take control of the situation. You mustn't lose your nerve or giggle. To pull this off successfully, you'll need a great deal of concentration and confidence. So, start as you mean to go on – focus!

Take the plunge
Push the door open slowly, and appear. Walk towards him with an air of such confidence you actually strut! Your

25

posture will speak volumes. Don't rush, or else you may trip or wobble. Be predatory and sure-footed as you stalk your prey. Move at a pace that you're comfortable with; this is your dance and your show.

Don't be fazed by anything. Lock into your fantasy character; she has never met this man before. He's a stranger to her, but it's her destiny to dance for him tonight. If she dances well, he may favour her …

Create the fantasy with your imagination and the way you look at your lover. Enjoy the process, not just the final result.

A magical experience

From the moment you appear, there should be an air of excitement and joy in the room. Both of you should be smiling. Enjoy the intimacy of this bonding experience. Create a magical atmosphere. Imagine your power as a fabulous glow that surrounds you both. You will light up the room with your confidence. Let him know you're in love …

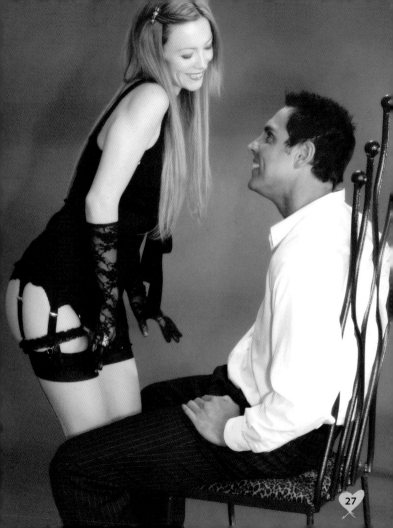

style matters

In this section I will explain how to make this dance effective, and I'll also suggest some easy ways to look confident and sexy. You don't need to be a great dancer; just remember to relax and enjoy yourself.

Of course, I couldn't write this book without sharing all the tricks of the trade! Everything I've learned about giving a stunning performance is here.

The golden rule is eye contact. If you can hold your lover in your gaze, he'll barely notice how you dance. What he won't fail to see is the magic and sensuality of the experience. Your confidence

28

and the fantasy will intoxicate you both.

Another key factor that can't be overemphasized is the importance of keeping it slow. There's no excuse for getting your feet in knots with this style of dancing. Your brain should be able to keep up with your feet, if not be slightly ahead of them.

I suggest that you don't let your lover touch you during your show – this is a rule that's strictly followed in the profession. Explain this to your partner when you make the date; it can add a whole new

dimension of excitement to the experience. After all, he's never met you before, has he!

However, you may wish to alter some of my rules, such as the 'no touch' policy. You must do whatever feels right to you.

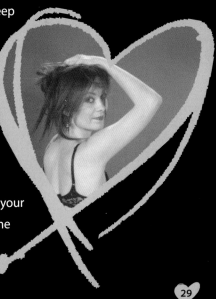

Eye contact is the key to making this one of the most incredible experiences you and your partner will share. The first thing he will notice will be your commitment. It's no good walking in and giggling, or not looking directly at him. Neither is it erotic if you instantly fall out of character and lose your nerve. This will make you seem uncomfortable and therefore will make him feel uncomfortable, too.

Remember that behaviour breeds behaviour, so be confident and look directly at your man with an enigmatic smile. This is the most important part of your performance. If he believes in you, he will feel confident enough to look at you and enjoy what you're doing. You may find that he seems to be looking only into your eyes.

Building a rapport

Slowly walk towards your lover. If his legs are crossed or closed, kneel down at his feet and gently push his knees apart to create a space for you to dance within. If his hands are on his lap or locked across his groin, move them to his

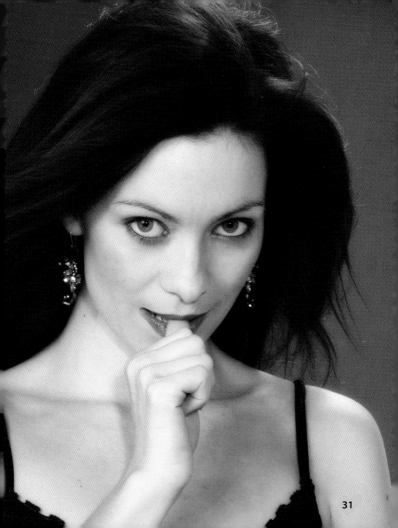

sides. And make sure he sits up straight.

With full eye contact, introduce yourself (or your fantasy character – see pages 88–9) slowly and explain to your man that he mustn't touch you or speak to you while you dance. If he tries to touch you, gently place his hands back by his sides. If he tries to speak to you, politely ignore him. For the time being, you do not speak his language.

Lead his gaze

During your performance, you can use eye contact to control your lover's gaze. As you undulate or sway your hips, cup your breasts in your hands. Look down at them, then back at him. This simple eye movement will lead his eye to the place you wish him to see.

Whatever dance moves you choose and whatever you wear, as long as you maintain eye contact as much as possible you will have the love of your life eating from the palm of your hand.

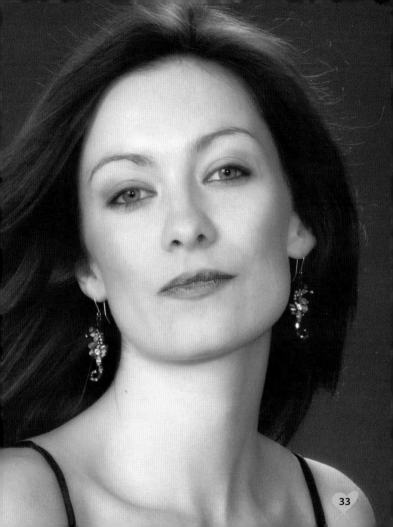

As you dance, as well as keeping your movement slow, try to make it flow. Find a hidden rhythm within the music, rather than moving to the dictated beat. Control your movement with every muscle and sinew in your body, including your brain!

By gently swaying and moving in an elegant, feminine way, you become hypnotic. You are in control. Allow yourself to relax and breathe gently. Hypnotize your lover with your magnetism. He will be transfixed by your beauty.

Where to parade

Always dance in front of your audience, never to the side. You're trying to create a sexual frisson, so always remain directly in line with his groin. Allow him to admire you from afar as well as up close. This is simulated sex

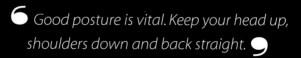

Good posture is vital. Keep your head up, shoulders down and back straight.

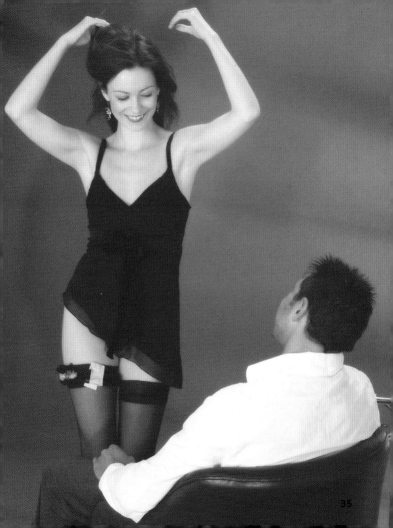

in dance form. You pull away, get close, pull away, get even closer …

Keep moving

Undulate your whole body, keeping your eyes on your man. This graceful movement is what connects together the dance moves that follow. You should have a beautiful expression on your face throughout the show. You may wink, smile and lick your lips, but never frown or look away from your audience.

If you have moments when your mind goes blank and you can't think what to do next, be still, strike a pose and look your man straight in the eye. Then slowly begin to undulate and parade again.

As you move, concentrate on keeping your neck elongated and your shoulders down. Your face should be on display; don't hide it behind hunched shoulders.

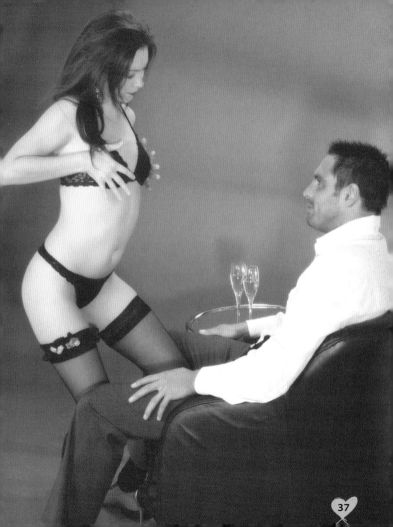

We all have a tendency to compartmentalize the figure; we say things like, 'Wow, that woman has lovely breasts,' or, 'Look at those legs,' or, 'She has hot lips,' or 'Look at that guy's ass!' But, deep down, unless you're a fetishist, if you love someone, you love everything about them, inside and out.

Showing off your best bits
With this style of dancing, the intention is to showcase all your assets in one go, to form a wonderful whole, finishing it off with large helpings of style, confidence and

character. Make your man fall in love with every part of you, all over again.

The way to draw attention to your assets, to invite your lover to appreciate them all, is to touch and stroke them. Your hands should trace a sensual trail from your hair, down your face and lips, over your breasts and across your body. Caress your buttocks and inner thighs. Using your hands rather than your voice, give him permission to look at and admire you.

Keep stroking yourself in this way throughout the

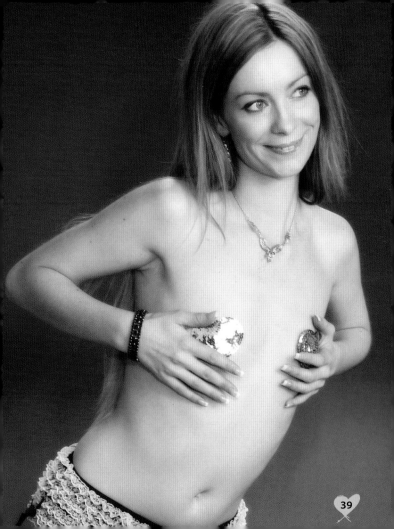

show. Give the impression that you are totally in love with yourself.

Armed and dangerous

Touching yourself will send potent signals to your partner, and will make him wish your hands were his hands. It will also send a subliminal message saying that you love, respect and admire your body, so he can feel free to do the same.

Be delicate with your touch. In Tantric philosophy, it is said that lovers should give each other a light massage before sexual congress. This will get the blood flowing through the capillaries and, therefore, will make you both more receptive to pleasure. Turn yourself on. Really enjoy the sensuousness of your own touch.

Remember also that it's alright for you to touch him. Gently stroke his hair, face, chest and legs. He will find this exciting, as he still mustn't touch you.

Don't feel ashamed to be sexy. Be proud of who you are.

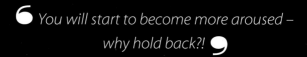

You will start to become more aroused – why hold back?!

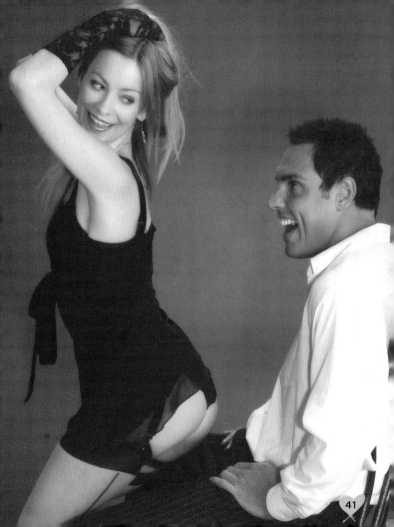

using props

If you find yourself naked too soon or simply wish to add something different to your routine, props are the answer.

Use your imagination, but don't use too many props in one show – you don't want to look like a circus performer.

Focus on being sensual and sexual, not on trying to juggle hats and boas.

Champagne

Champagne or sparkling wine can be used in many different ways. For instance, if your breasts are uncovered, take a full mouthful as you dance, then allow a gentle, controlled stream to flow from your lips, over your nipples and down your tummy. Turn around, look over your shoulder and trickle the remainder over your back and bottom. Then rub it all over yourself erotically as you continue to dance.

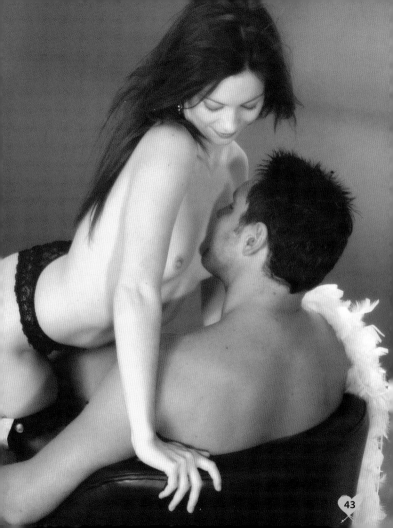

Sounds tricky, I know, but with practice it can be done! And it's worth persevering until you get the knack, because the glistening liquid on your skin will look and feel amazing. If you're not feeling very wealthy or have carpeted floors, this trick works equally well with water.

When you've mastered the basic technique, you could try this variation: stand over your lover and trickle the liquid over your nipples and into his mouth! If you wish to keep things more straightforward, simply pass the liquid from mouth to mouth.

Some of the classics

There are many items that make great props. Here are some of my favourites.

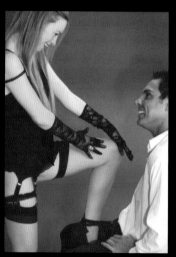

Nipple tassels are great if you want to surprise your man. Wear them underneath your bra so they're hidden.

When you reveal them, he'll be thrilled. You don't need to be able to twirl them because they look fabulous, anyway.

Feather boa This is one of the best. Don't keep it on all the way through; wear it as you walk in, then take it off almost straight away, leaving it where you can easily pick it up again. When you remove your bra or knickers later on, you could use the feather boa to cover yourself, then slowly pull it off as the music closes.

Long gloves look fabulous if you leave them on throughout the performance. Black ones are flattering for pale skin,

white or bright colours look fabulous on darker skin.

Chair or stool This is another popular choice. Use it to lean on as well as sit on. If it doesn't weigh much, you can move it around as you dance, so that it's in the correct position for your next move. For some great tips on dancing with a chair, watch the movie *Cabaret*.

Hat Remove this last of all, and use it to cover your breasts or groin. Then, just before the music finishes, move it away slowly to reveal yourself. At the very end, place your hat on your lover's head.

dance moves

There are many ways to move erotically, and in this section I shall teach you the most common ones. The moves themselves are simple; the skill is in linking them together to create a dance routine that will stay on your lover's mind long after the music stops!

The hip movements you will learn are incredibly potent to watch. They involve the lower back, which is where *Kundalini*, sexual energy, is stored. Moving in this way subliminally indicates that we're preparing for sex.

Be inspired

The moves I've included here are purely suggestions

designed to inspire you to come up with your own. Invest in a full-length mirror for your bedroom, and use it to try out ideas and to check out what moves suit your body. If possible, do this whenever you have time to yourself.

Try to develop a new persona – a fantasy character – and call upon her to guide you. Attempt to evoke the temple dancer within. Imagine you've been practising the ancient arts of love for many millennia. Project your fantasy on to your partner through the windows of his soul – his eyes.

Imagine simulating sex in a graceful and flowing way. Show your lover how slowly and beautifully you can dance. Recreate some of the movements involved

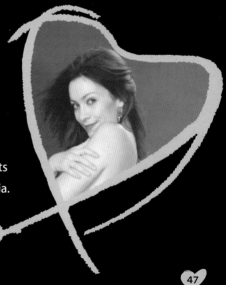

in making love. You can do this from a distance, close up, on a chair, standing up, astride him or kneeling in front of him on the floor.

Attention to detail
Throughout your show, whatever you do, each move should flow seamlessly into the next. Try to emulate the flawless movements of a snake or a big cat.

As you move, don't forget about your facial expressions – your face should reflect love and passion throughout the performance. Stick to moves that you can achieve without having to concentrate too hard; you don't want to overstretch yourself and end up frowning. Continue to look sexy and engrossed in what you're doing all the way through. Stay in control of your body and your mind.

Make sure you're always moving. When you're not performing a specific dance move, simply sway and undulate your hips.

Experimentation
The moves in this chapter aren't intended to be a list of things to do. Just choose the ones you like best, or try a few different ones each time you dance for your lover. You don't need to use them all in one show.

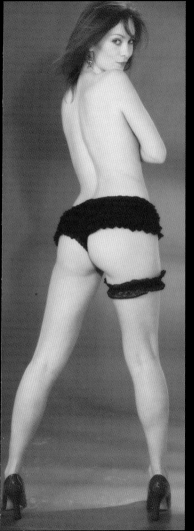

When you're alone, practise your chosen moves in front of the chair where your partner will be seated for your show. This will give you a sense of the space you'll have, and help to put things into perspective.

It is important that you breathe deeply as you dance. And, above all, remember these three rules: eye contact; shoulders down; keep it slow!

the walk

When you walk towards or away from your lover, move like a jungle cat. Arch your back and push your breasts out. Keep the shoulders down and allow your arms to move naturally, following the suggestions given in Arm Movement (*see pages 38–40*).

Enjoy the parade. Have fun watching your man watching you. Seeing someone walking with style and panache is hypnotizing. Always strut – be the sex kitten you've always wanted to be! Dazzle yourself with your cheeky confidence. Feel the magic in the air around you. Let it sizzle, baby!

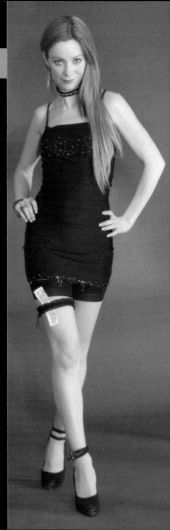

the body wave

As you stand facing your lover, imagine you're a snake being charmed from its basket. This is a slow wave up through the body from the ankle to the breasts. Keep your feet together, shoulders down and your back straight or arched. Undulate your pelvis forwards and backwards so your movement ripples through all the muscles in your abdomen and lower thighs.

When I was working as a professional dancer, I found that undulating my body in this way gave me a fantastic flat stomach with loads of definition.

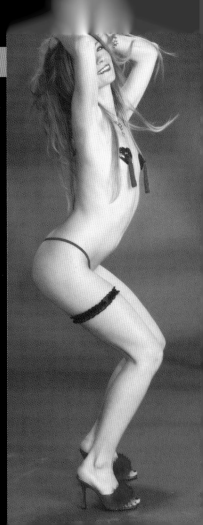

the figure eight

With your feet together and your knees slightly bent, begin to circle your hips. Push the left hip, then the right, out to the side, to make a figure eight with your pelvis. Don't jerk the hips; aim for a flowing, subtle movement. Imagine you have a paintbrush attached to your knickers and you're painting a figure eight on the floor.

As you do this, caress your breasts and hair with your arms and hands.

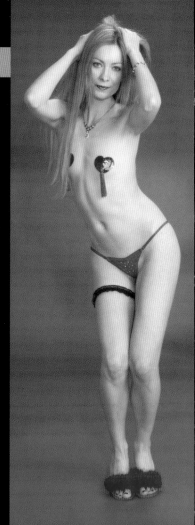

the circle

Again, with your feet together and knees slightly bent, focus on that paintbrush and paint a big circle on the floor. Push your hips out as you do this to make a large circle. This move is fantastic for emphasizing the female shape.

Running your hands through your hair is really sexy, and if you mess it up, hey presto, you've changed your image again!

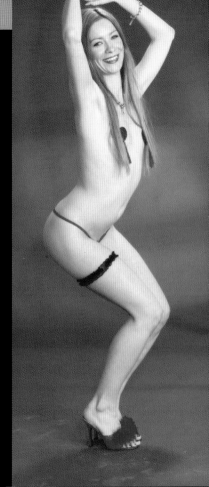

the marilyn pose

This move works well either standing a little way away from your audience or right up close.

Stand up straight and, still with your feet together, shift your weight from one foot to the other, bending the knees slightly as you do so. Bend forwards with your knees straight and push your breasts together, either with your hands or upper arms. Your breasts should be level with your lover's eyes. Slowly stand up straight again and undulate your hips or sway.

54

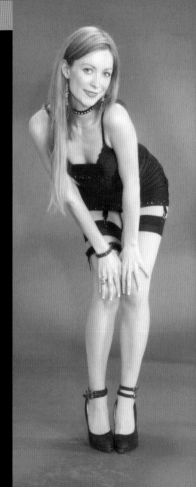

the shimmy

The shimmy is a variation on the figure eight (*see page 52*). So, keep your feet together, and as you repeat the figure-eight movement with your hips, bend your knees as far as is comfortable. Don't let your heels lift off the floor. Then, still moving your hips, rise back up to a standing position.

This is a lovely, slow movement that, like the body wave (*see page 51*), resembles a snake being charmed from a basket.

❝ *Dance slowly and hypnotize your lover with your control.* **❞**

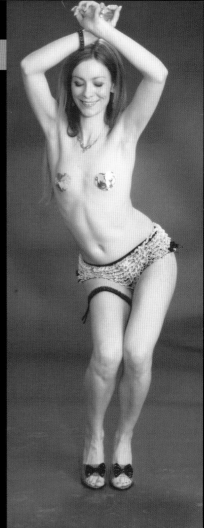

the grinding circle

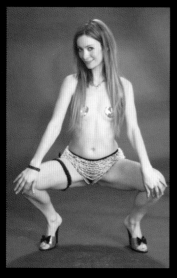

Stand about 60 centimetres (2 feet) from your partner, with your feet slightly more than hip-width apart and your toes turned out. With your hips, begin to draw that circle again, keeping your back arched. Now, slowly bend your knees and grind down as far as is comfortable, then up again, continually undulating your hips and dancing erotically.

It's really important to keep your back arched and upright. If you lean forward, you risk impersonating a Sumo wrestler!

❝ *Keep your shoulders relaxed and down – don't hunch!* ❞

As I've said, lap dancing is about showing off all your assets, so remember to turn around occasionally. For the best effect, turn slowly – your lover should barely notice.

When you practise, work out which direction is most natural for you to turn in. And don't be overly concerned with how you do it; just take small steps and aim to make the turn blend into and become part of your dance. Keep circling your hips, and remember your arm movements. As far as possible, try to keep your lover in your gaze as you turn.

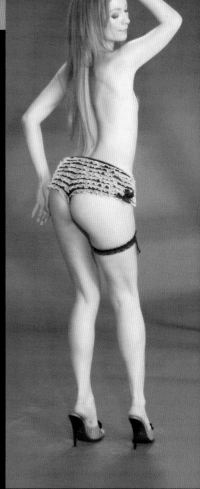

Turn your back to your audience and, with straight legs, bend forwards slightly, look back at him coquettishly and stroke or lightly slap your bottom. I guarantee this will make him smile.

Alternatively, still with you back to him, gently sway from your ankles, opening your leg gradually. Slowly, bend over s that your bottom is brazenly pointing at your man. Bend one knee to the side and straighten the other out to the other side. Glide your hand up the straight leg and raise your head over the corresponding shoulder to look back at him. Slap your bottom hard. Repeat on the other side.

the lap dance grind

Gracefully dance yourself into the triangle made by your lover's open legs, and stand with your back to him, your feet together. Make sure you're as close to the chair as possible.

Now bend your knees, keeping your back straight, and gently put your hands on your partner's knees. Lower your bottom towards his lap so that you can just feel his crotch on your skin. Then, keeping your hands on his knees for support, grind down gently, moving your hips in a circular or forward-and-backward motion.

Look over your shoulder at your man while you do this, if you can. This is a little tricky, though!

Take extra care whenever you go near his groin. If you hurt him, he'll never trust you to dance for him again!

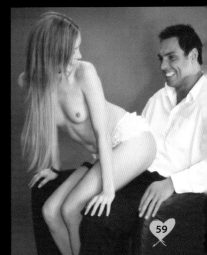

the breast stroke

Every woman has her own personal scent that collects in between her breasts, no matter what size they are or what perfume she wears. It's a potent aphrodisiac. So this step is guaranteed to get your lover going!

Move closely into the space between his knees. Standing with your legs straight, gently lean forward and place your hands on either side of the chair. Once you have a firm hold, push your breasts towards his face; his nose should be nestled in your cleavage. For added effect, try brushing from side to side and stroking the end of his nose with your bra or nipple. Keep moving in a provocative way throughout.

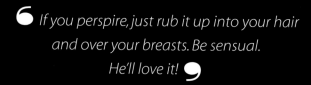

If you perspire, just rub it up into your hair and over your breasts. Be sensual. He'll love it!

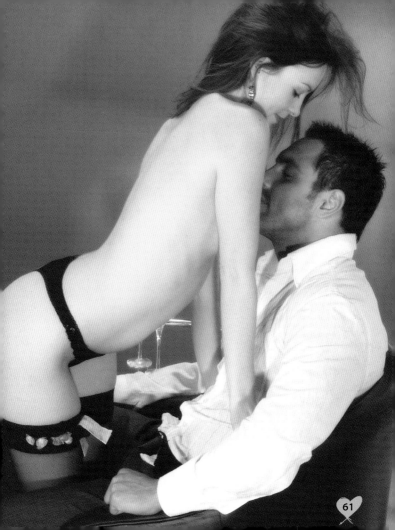

knee strokes

Facing your partner, stand in between his legs, as close to the chair as you can. Place your knees in the space between his crotch and the edge of the chair. Gently put a slight pressure against his groin with your knees. Lean towards him and blow gently into his ear or on his face. You could even exchange a mouthful of wine with him or pour champagne from your nipples into his mouth.

As a variation, try this: stand up facing your lover, then catch one of his knees between your knees and gently rub up and down his thigh. This is a fabulous sensation. Ask him to do it to you sometime!

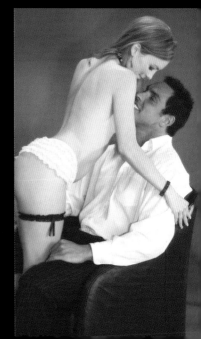

the body slide

This is a lovely move, but you'll need to use your own judgement as to whether your partner is able to take your weight!

Standing between your lover's thighs, lean forwards and put your hands on the back of the chair for support. Put one knee on each of his thighs, then lift your torso, slide your knees into the space in front of his crotch (careful here!) and slide, slowly, all the way down his body until you're kneeling on the floor in front of him.

To get up off the floor, use your lover's knees for support and stand up sexily – bring your bottom up first, then flick your hair in his face as you raise your upper body.

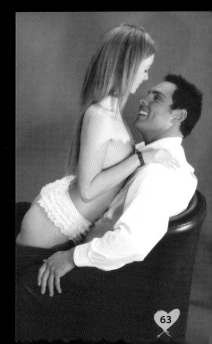

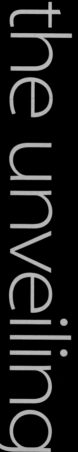

the unveiling

It's time to put all your knowledge to good use! The following pages contain an example of a dance routine using the moves you've learned. It also incorporates the undressing, so you'll see how all aspects of the performance work together.

The secret to unveiling, or stripping, erotically is not to rush. This is striptease – 'tease' being the operative word. The quest to uncover a secret usually makes the hidden truth all the more satisfying.

Enjoy every moment. Drop a shoulder strap, then give nothing more away for a minute or two. Be provocative. Show him a flash of breast by lowering your bra for a moment, then covering up again.

I recommend that you dance to two pieces of music. Towards the end of the first song, slowly take off your dress. During the second song, allow time for your lover to appreciate you in your underwear before you remove anything else. You're now a different woman – you've changed your image again.

If you decide to go nude, you may need a third song. It's important that you learn to judge where each song ends, so practise your dance and get to know your music.

Remember: it's the way you undress, not the *fact* that you're undressing, that makes this dance arousing. Don't get naked and prance around all the way through – that's another ritual altogether.

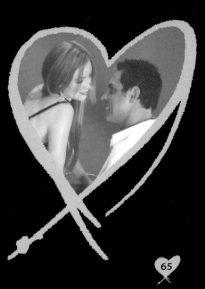

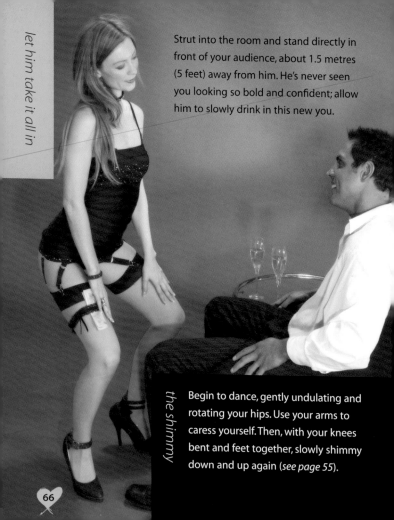

Strut into the room and stand directly in front of your audience, about 1.5 metres (5 feet) away from him. He's never seen you looking so bold and confident; allow him to slowly drink in this new you.

the shimmy

Begin to dance, gently undulating and rotating your hips. Use your arms to caress yourself. Then, with your knees bent and feet together, slowly shimmy down and up again (*see page 55*).

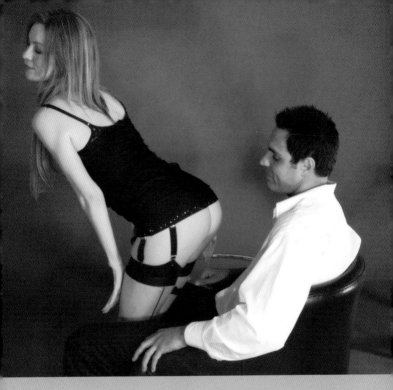

Keeping your eyes on your lover, turn around slowly; let him see every angle of your body. With your back to him, put your feet together and bend forwards as far as you can, keeping your legs straight. Aim to touch your toes. Slowly stand up and turn to face him. He's now seen how magical you look. Whenever you have your back to your lover, push your bum out and arch your back.

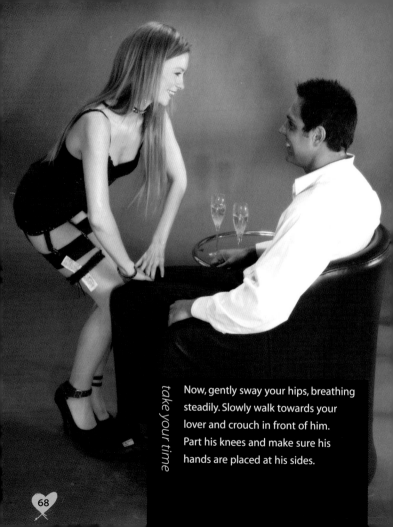

take your time

Now, gently sway your hips, breathing steadily. Slowly walk towards your lover and crouch in front of him. Part his knees and make sure his hands are placed at his sides.

68

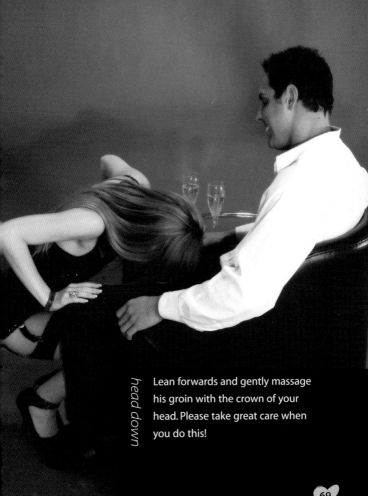

head down

Lean forwards and gently massage his groin with the crown of your head. Please take great care when you do this!

69

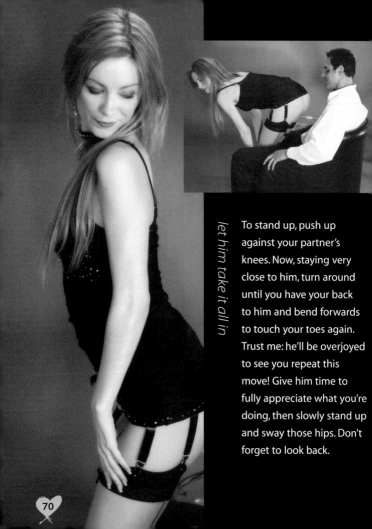

let him take it all in

To stand up, push up against your partner's knees. Now, staying very close to him, turn around until you have your back to him and bend forwards to touch your toes again. Trust me: he'll be overjoyed to see you repeat this move! Give him time to fully appreciate what you're doing, then slowly stand up and sway those hips. Don't forget to look back.

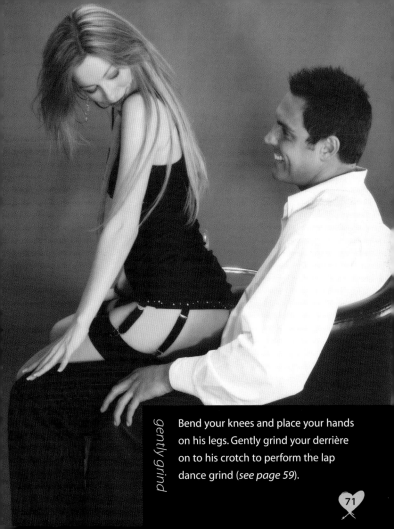

gently grind

Bend your knees and place your hands on his legs. Gently grind your derrière on to his crotch to perform the lap dance grind (*see page 59*).

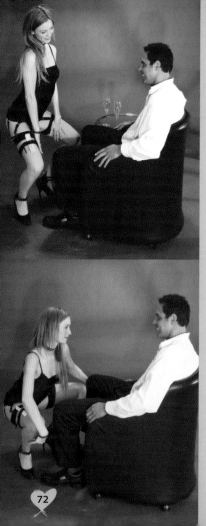

Stand up straight and walk a little further away – never stay close to your audience for very long. Now, turn to face him and open your legs to slightly more than hip-width apart. Your toes should be turned outwards and your knees bent. Begin to rotate your hips – do not lean forwards. Only bend as far as you can before you start to feel yourself lean. In between circling your hips, bump up and down a couple of times (simulating what you'll be doing later!). Then stand up straight and slide your feet back together. For details of this move in full, see page 56.

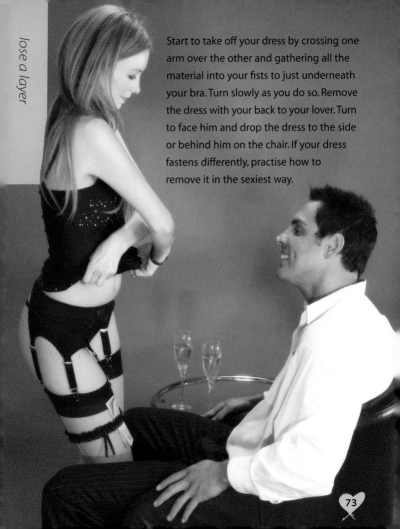

Start to take off your dress by crossing one arm over the other and gathering all the material into your fists to just underneath your bra. Turn slowly as you do so. Remove the dress with your back to your lover. Turn to face him and drop the dress to the side or behind him on the chair. If your dress fastens differently, practise how to remove it in the sexiest way.

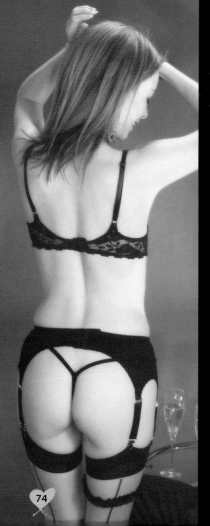

flaunt your goods

Now you've done the difficult bit – the dress is off. Dance and enjoy yourself. Walk away from him again so that he can see this lovely, scantily clad creature you've become. Face him and caress yourself all over as you undulate your hips hypnotically. The worst thing you could do now is rush.

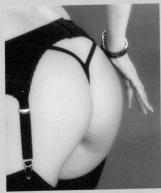

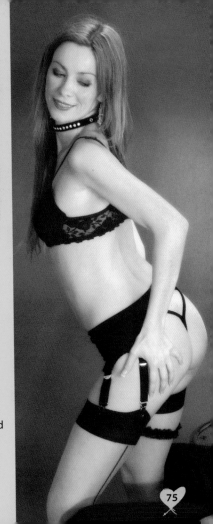

slap your bum

Lean forwards and push your cleavage together with your hands. As you straighten up again, turn and bend forwards with your legs apart. Bending one knee, lunge to the side. Stroke your hand up your leg, look over your shoulder and slap your bum. Repeat to the other side. Stand up straight and turn to face your lover, swaying your hips as you do so.

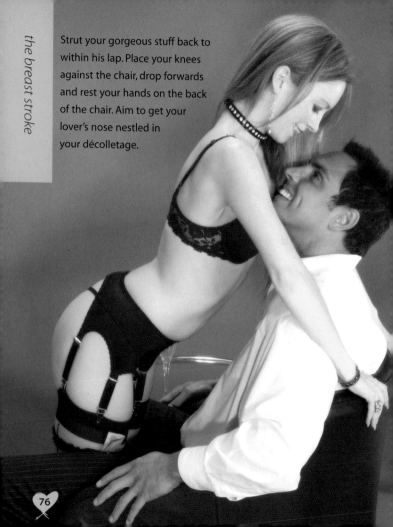

Strut your gorgeous stuff back to within his lap. Place your knees against the chair, drop forwards and rest your hands on the back of the chair. Aim to get your lover's nose nestled in your décolletage.

If he's strong enough to take your weight, you could try this: press your whole body on to his and allow yourself to slide down over him until you are kneeling on the floor. Alternatively, simply push against the chair to stand upright, then shimmy down and kneel between his knees.

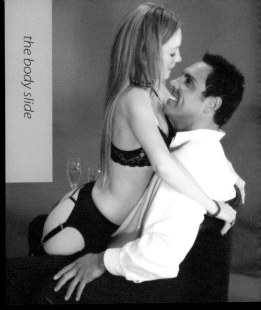

the body slide

let it all go!

Put both hands on your lover's knees, push your breasts onto his crotch and, gently but firmly, massage him with them. Then, leave one hand on his knee and bend backwards, letting the other arm fly back with a flourish. Let your head fall back – the aim here is to look as though you're in the throes of ecstasy. Try to circle your pelvis as well, or do pelvic thrusts up towards your lover.

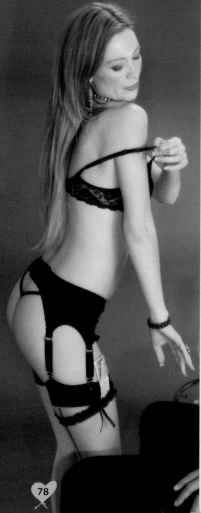

Return to a crouching position and push up against your partner's knees to enable you to stand. Stay as close to him as you can, and dance hypnotically between his knees. Now, turn until you're in profile. Using the opposite hand, slowly pull down your bra strap and glide your arm through to remove it completely. Turn to face your lover and lean forwards to stroke his face.

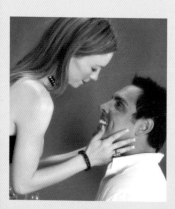

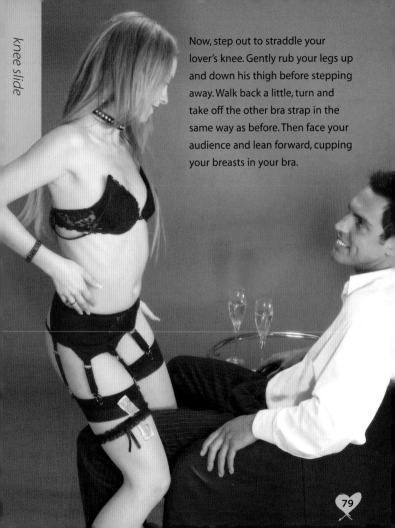

Now, step out to straddle your lover's knee. Gently rub your legs up and down his thigh before stepping away. Walk back a little, turn and take off the other bra strap in the same way as before. Then face your audience and lean forward, cupping your breasts in your bra.

79

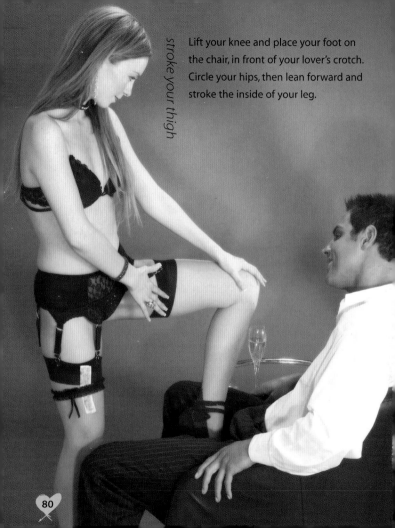

stroke your thigh

Lift your knee and place your foot on the chair, in front of your lover's crotch. Circle your hips, then lean forward and stroke the inside of your leg.

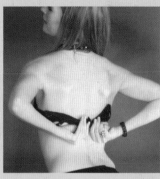

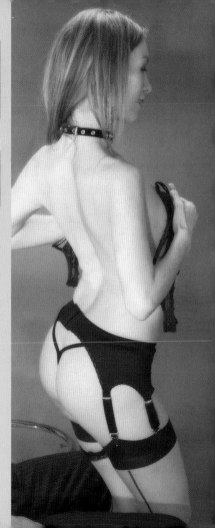

the big tease

Walk away and turn your back to him. Undo your bra but hold it in place. Turn to face him and dance provocatively as you drop your bra to one side. Don't let him see your breasts yet. Tease him. Let him have a peak at a nipple through your fingers, then turn away and put your hands into your hair. Turn back again, breasts hidden. Tantalize him like this for as long as you wish!

Very, very slowly, reveal your breasts. If you have enough music left, continue to dance and caress yourself. Repeat the dance moves that seemed to delight your lover the most!

Don't linger too long after your show – just long enough to offer your garter to him, perhaps. Hopefully, he'll know what to do …

making your exit

As soon as you have finished dancing, cover your breasts and groin (if you're naked) with your hands. Stand still, facing your audience. Keep smiling and look to see where your clothes are. They should either be behind his shoulders or to the side of him on the chair.

Walk towards your man, shoulders down, back straight, still covering yourself with your hands. Pick up your clothes quickly, and hold them close to your body.

Another new you

Just before you turn to leave, say, 'Thank you'. Then, immediately turn and walk away, slowly but surely.

Go to a different room so that you can get dressed out of sight. I strongly recommend that you have another costume ready to wear. Retouch your make-up and hair and apply a little fresh perfume. Then return to your admiring audience.

Have a few drinks together, have a laugh,

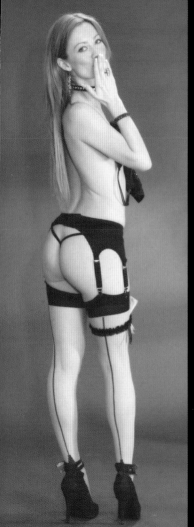

do whatever you wish to do … But, who is this new girl beside him? Where did the other girl go? This girl has a different costume on – she must be a different person … Is she? Maybe he'll buy another dance.

❝ Once the music stops, leave quickly – preserve the mystery. ❞

the fantasy

When I dance for my lover I choose different characters to be for the duration of the show. In this section I shall introduce you to one of my fantasy characters, Phoenix, who I hope will inspire you to create your own persona. Remember: you can be anyone you want to be for the entire evening but, whoever you are, be dazzling!

I get asked all kinds of questions by the girls who come to my dance classes. If you have a query, you may find the answer in Your Questions Answered (*see pages 92–3*). There is plenty of information here that should help you if you lack confidence or feel a bit bewildered by it all.

Dancing erotically for your lover is like role play, and you may find it helpful to take a look at Confessions of a Lap Dancer (*see pages 94–5*) to get into the mind of a professional. I thought it would be fun to introduce you to some of the characters and situations that you would encounter in the clubs, so you can perform your role realistically! If you wish to just be yourself, however, then that's fine, too.

It's my wish that, after reading this section of the book, you'll feel totally prepared to put on a great show. I want you to relax and enjoy this experience to the full.

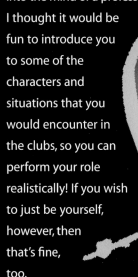

creating your fantasy character

Give yourself an alter ego – create a fantasy. Unleash that confident, sexy part of your character that doesn't get enough airplay.

Your fantasy name

It's imperative that you feel beautiful and worthy of admiration throughout this dance, so choose a fabulous name. Use only a single name.

Panther, Juliet, Luscious, Flame, Moon, Trixie …

Bond with your character

You may fantasize about being a lap dancer, or you may wish to be a goddess. Whatever your preference, a great way to explore and get to know your fantasy character is to write a free-flowing page or two about her. What's her

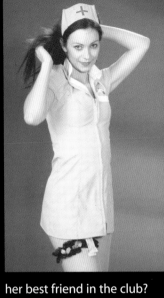

You can be anyone you like, tonight.

If you wish, you can use a different character each time you perform, or keep with the same one. It's up to you.

Set the scene

When you make the date with your lover, tell him who it is that will be dancing for him.

her best friend in the club? And the name of the bitch? What's the boss like? Does your character have a day job? Is she a reporter from a tabloid newspaper trying to get an inside scoop on the girls? Does she fancy one of the customers? Is she a spy? Fall in love with your new self.

Say, 'Hey, honey, that's the night Phoenix is working', or 'Angel would like to see you on Friday night; she's a great dancer – you'll like her a lot.'

You don't have to follow my script to the letter, but do try to add to the anticipation in this way. He'll love every moment of it, I can assure you.

'My name is Phoenix. I come from a faraway land where the forests twinkle at night. The forest people collect there and dance, sing and make merry. We love to make love with those we choose. There are no dangers. We are free. There is no prejudice. We have no concept of hatred or evil, except what we've learned from history's mistakes. We are all loved.

'I'm a strong woman, although I've made some bad choices when it comes to men – but this makes me wise and powerful. I always turn adversity into triumph.

I'm motivated by health and fitness, and I'm gorgeous. I ooze sex from every pore because I understand human nature; I adore people and they adore me. I also have a magical, mystical quality, which is my spirituality. I have the spark of the goddess within.

'My passion is to dance. My imagination soars as I glide through the beautiful, glittering landscape. I love my life, but, when I dance, I'm *in* love with my life.

'I am passionate about dressing up in beautiful costumes. I become a truly

90

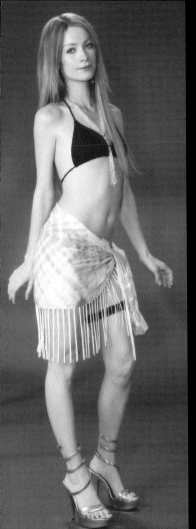

stunning creature as I prepare. I dance in the forest. There are lights and glitter everywhere, but I imagine they are made of fairy dust. My soul mate watches me secretly from afar, waiting for the right moment to present himself.

'I weave magical spells wherever I go. My eyes can penetrate the iciest stare and melt the hardest heart. I can solve everything with love and compassion. I have been sent from a distant future to bring spirituality, peace, love and humanity to everyone I meet.

'My mission here begins with love and ends in love. I am Phoenix.'

Your questions answered

Am I degrading myself by stripping for my partner?
No way. You're giving him a delightful treat. This is a bonding ritual and a secret to share. It's a wonderful night in for you both to enjoy. If you feel degraded in any way, I suggest you talk to your partner before you make the date. I'm sure he will put your mind at rest. Try to have fun. And remember: giving goes both ways. Make sure he treats you to something nice, as well, sometime.

What if he laughs?
A little laughter is OK – this is supposed to be fun, after all! But, if he laughs *at* you rather than *with* you, perhaps your performance is more comical than sensuous! Did you give him sufficient warning? Have you followed my instructions on eye contact? If you're doing everything right and he still laughs, then frankly, my dear,

you shouldn't give a damn about him anyway.

What if I giggle?
Your fantasy character probably wouldn't giggle. She might smile beguilingly and purr deep down in her chest at the thought of what might come later. Her eyes may even light up at the sight of this handsome mortal! If you giggle, you'll just appear nervous.

What if I forget what to do?
Just keep moving gently and turning occasionally until something comes to mind. You don't have to include specific moves in your routine in order to entertain your lover.

I find eye contact difficult. What should I do?
Try to be brave, and hold your lover in that magnetic, magical, mischievous gaze of yours. If you

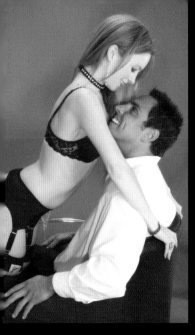

it faze you. Carry on and be brilliant, regardless.

What if my costume gets tangled or stuck?
Turn your back to your audience, devote your attention to the problem and quickly sort it out. If this doesn't work, improvise! To prevent this from happening, always rehearse using the clothes you will wear on the night.

Is it better to go topless or completely nude?
It's entirely up to you. Perhaps you could just go topless the first time, then next time go nude – he'll be blown away by the surprise!

Could my lover be naked?
It's totally up to you – you're in charge.

absolutely can't do this, then wear a mask that covers only your eyes. But, be warned: this may restrict your vision slightly and could make dancing a bit more difficult.

What if I make a mistake?
This is a slow dance, so with any luck you won't have any problems. If you do trip or stumble, don't let

confessions of a lap dancer

The people you meet, the things you see –
it's another world!

The Fans As long as they don't have your phone number, they're the perks of the job.

The Old Fools They're suckers for flattery and are desperate to believe that a beautiful young dancer would fancy them. Play along with their fantasy and they'll buy lots of dances – they're paying to feel young again.

The Millionaires They can be incredibly generous, or equally mean; hygienically challenged with a penchant for toupees, or gorgeous well-mannered gentlemen. Money amplifies the virtues *and* the faults.

The House Mother Officially, she's employed to help you with costume

problems and to organize the rota. Really she's there to undermine and intimidate you because you don't give her a big enough tip at the end of the night.

The Boyfriends What boyfriends? Going out with an erotic dancer can be quite intimidating. There was no one special in my life until I retired.

The Camaraderie I've made some of the best friends of my life as a dancer. Genuine performers are the most amazingly beautiful people, inside and out, that you'll ever have the honour to know.

The Highs and Lows Plug into this reality and taste the disappointment